HEALTHY GREEN SMOOTHIES

50 Easy Recipes that will Change Your Life

Duc Vuong, M.D.

ISBN-13: 978-0692980743

ISBN-10: 0692980741

Published by HappyStance Publishing. Interior formatting and cover design by Tony Loton of LOTONtech Limited, www.lotontech.com.

The information contained in this book is not designed to replace or take the place of any form of medicine or professional medical advice. The information in this book has been provided for educational and entertainment purposes only. The information contained in this book has been compiled from sources deemed reliable, and it is accurate to the best of the Author's knowledge; however, the Author cannot guarantee its accuracy and validity and cannot be held liable for any errors or omissions. Changes are periodically made to this book. You must consult your doctor or get professional medical advice before using any of the suggested remedies, techniques, or information in this book. Upon using the information contained in this book, you agree to hold harmless the Author from and against any damages, costs, and expenses, including any legal fees potentially resulting from the application of any of the information provided by this guide. This disclaimer applies to any damages or injury caused by the use and application, whether directly or indirectly, of any advice or information presented, whether for breach of contract, tort, negligence, personal injury, criminal intent, or under any other cause of action. You agree to accept all risks of using the information presented inside this book. You need to consult a professional medical practitioner in order to ensure you are both able and healthy enough to participate in this program. Although Dr. Vuong is a medical doctor, he is most likely not your doctor, and this book in no way creates a doctor-patient relationship between you, the reader, and him.

Contents

Foreword

A pulsing buzz fills the room at 5:15 a.m. The dog stirs and so does the cat, but not Sabrina. Sabrina can hardly drag her eyes open. With a sigh halfway to a grunt of effort, she rolls herself over and blindly probes for her alarm clock. Lethargic, heavy arms grope around for what seems like hours before landing on the snooze button. Groggily, Sabrina blinks the fog from her eyes and struggles to sit up.

It's like even sitting up gets harder every day, she thinks while letting out a sigh. *Maybe it's a good sign that today is the day* .

The day she means is the start of a new way of life. Weeks before, she found a recipe book for green smoothies and laid plans to begin a healthier lifestyle. Her boyfriend bought her a fancy smoothies blender and new tumbler glasses for Valentine's Day. She has been including the ingredients in her groceries but, plagued with lethargy, her plans have stalled .

She dresses quickly, eagerly anticipating a change of her morning routine. Waking up her tablet, she looks over recipes on her way to the kitchen. Settling on an Orange and Avocado Twist, she readies her blender and raids the refrigerator for ingredients. Peeling the fruit and pitting the avocado is a pretty quick affair, so Sabrina is loading the blender within minutes. She muses on how much simpler it is to work a blender than the time-sensitive multitasking of her usual eggs, sausage and toast.

She checks the blender and notes the uniform light green of its contents. From today forward, this will be the color of breakfast. Pouring half into a glass, she looks it over. It is smooth, green and uniformly mixed so she is confident she has made it properly. Tentatively at first, Sabrina tastes it. The smoothie has a light, creamy texture and tastes much sweeter and fruitier than she expected. It goes down easily, soon leaving her with nothing more than an empty cup and a satisfied grin. She pours the rest into a capped bottle and stows it away with her drive to work.

I think I like this new morning routine! Sabrina says to herself.

Clean-up is a cinch, much easier than scrubbing a greasy pan. Sabrina finishes her preparations before work and checks the time on her cell phone as she heads out the door. Her new morning routine has saved her over ten minutes. She gets to work even earlier because the time she saved keeps her ahead of morning traffic. Arriving at work in good spirits, she settles in at her desk, ready for whatever the day has in store.

Introduction

What is a Smoothie?

What is Sabrina consuming for breakfast now? A green smoothie. A smoothie is a thick blended beverage with shake-like consistency, normally pureed in an emulsifier, which is a more powerful blender, specifically designed for creating smoothies. The ingredients include a myriad of fruits and / or vegetables, as well as a liquid such as water, fruit juice, vegetable juice, milk, or even yogurt.

Traditionally, most smoothies consist of three parts: some type of liquid (often called the "base" of the smoothie), an assortment of fruits and/or vegetables, and ice. If frozen fruit or vegetables are used, the cool temperature can be achieved without using ice.

Categories of Smoothies

- **Fruit Smoothies:** A smoothie made from fruits, specifically for their sweet flavor.
- **Green Smoothies:** Smoothies typically dark green in color due to their use of dark vegetable greens such as spinach.
- **Healthy Smoothies:** Any smoothie whose aim is to optimize the amount of nutritional content , with the goal of replacing supplements and providing all of one's daily recommended vitamins and macro-nutrients in a natural form.
- **Weight Loss Smoothies:** These typically exclude any added sugar (with the aim of minimizing the overall glycemic load of the smoothie), and often contain healthy fats such as flax seed or almond butter to help satiate one's appetite. Caffeine based stimulants like green tea or coffee can also be added which further promote weight loss by both increasing metabolism and reducing appetite.

- **Dessert Smoothies:** Dessert smoothies typically contain added sugar or fat in the form of ice cream or syrups (many recipe books call for smoothies with either added sugar or dairy products) creating a dessert like beverage, which in many cases, tastes identical to a shake.

Why Drink Green Smoothies?

Green Smoothies are densely nutritious. This is the secret that Sabrina is embracing in her new lifestyle, and one you should too! The foods we consume need to be either NUTRITIOUS or NON - NUTRITIOUS. No more labels of "good," "bad," "low-calorie" or "low fat."

By combining high-nutrient vegetables with fruit, the result is a sweet and tasty drink with high amounts of vitamins and minerals. These ingredients are good for the skin and bones, reduce cravings and increase your energy throughout the day. Green smoothies can be used as a snack throughout the day or even replace a meal. Smoothies also have more fiber than processed foods such as juices by using whole fruit and vegetables.

As long as you have an emulsifying blender, smoothies are fast and easy to make. There are several brands of emulsifiers. Nutribullet, NutriNinja, and Vitamix are probably the most recognized brands. Because clean up is so easy, they can save you time and effort in the mornings, enabling you to sleep in later or perform other tasks more easily. Children of all ages love to drink smoothies, and smoothies can be a tool to teach healthy eating habits. By providing a single source of numerous nutrients, smoothies are an ideal breakfast for growing children, as opposed to sugary cereals. Smoothies can be taken to school or work, can be made as a healthy lunch alternative, or served as a cold treat on hot summer days. With a snack so versatile, how can you not want to have one?

These recipes are simple to make. The ingredient amounts can be altered to suit your particular tastes. For example, if you don't like kale, you can use less of it or even substitute spinach for it. Lactose intolerant? Then you can substitute with soy or almond milk. Something out of season? You can try a different fruit of similar texture. The possibilities are really endless.

Smoothies simplify your life. Find two or three go-to recipes for weekday mornings and use the weekends to experiment with more exotic recipes. Personally, my mornings start with a smoothie consisting of spinach, small banana, frozen blueberries, frozen cherries, water, and local honey. I do not measure the ingredients.

1. Banana Burst

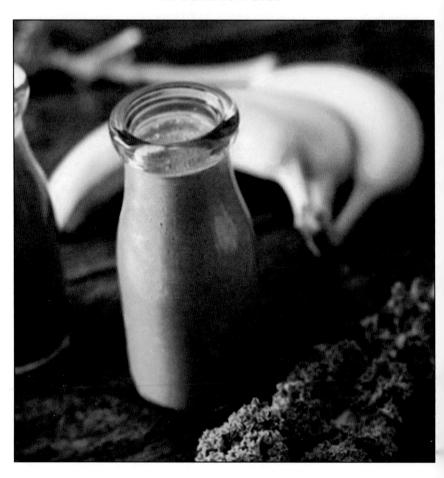

Get your day started with this simple recipe that packs not only great taste but also an extra punch of energy. Apples and bananas are the two most popular fruit in North America, and any variety is acceptable. Add in some fresh kale leaves, which have been popularly cultivated since men wore togas, and you can safely say this smoothie is for the "cool kids' table".

Prep Time : 5 min, Serve : 2

Ingredients

- 4 bananas, cut and frozen. If using fresh bananas, you will add some ice cubes.
- 2 large green apples, cored
- 4 tablespoons flax seed
- 2 cups kale, washed and chopped
- 2 cups coconut water to desired texture

Directions

Add all ingredients into a blender and blend on high speed until smooth .

Why This is Good For You

- Low in saturated fat
- No cholesterol
- Very low in sodium
- High in dietary fiber
- High in manganese
- High in magnesium
- Very high in vitamin C

Nutrition Facts

Calories 308, Calories from Fat 116, Total Fat 12.9g, Saturated Fat 1.3g, Trans Fat 0.0g, Cholesterol 0mg, Sodium 12mg, Potassium 840mg, Total Carbohydrates 46.1g, Dietary Fiber 14.8g, Sugars 20.1g, Protein 7.5g.

2. Orange and Avocado Twist

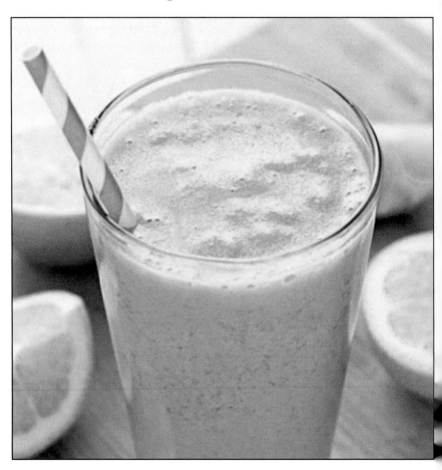

Wake yourself up with this simple yet thickset smoothie. It gets its body from meaty fruits such as bananas, oranges and an avocado. Being on the high-end of calories among our recipes, this choice can be a meal substitute in a pinch.

Prep Time: 5 min, Serve: 2

Ingredients

- 1 avocado, peeled with pit removed
- 2 bananas, cut and frozen. If using fresh bananas, you will need to add a few ice cubes.
- 2 large oranges, peeled
- 2 cups kale, washed
- 2 cups water to desired texture

Directions

Put all ingredients into a blender and blend on high speed until smooth. Enjoy your smoothie.

Why This is Good For You

- No cholesterol
- Low in sodium
- High in calcium
- High in dietary fiber
- High in potassium
- Very high in vitamin A
- High in vitamin B6
- Very high in vitamin C
- High in vitamin E

Nutrition Facts

Calories 499, Calories from Fat 270, Total Fat 30.0g, Saturated Fat 3.9g, Trans Fat 0.0g, Cholesterol 0mg, Sodium 212mg, Potassium 2031mg, Total Carbohydrates 60.5g, Dietary Fiber 20.3g, Sugars 27.5g, Protein 8.6g.

3. Blueberry Flourish Smoothie

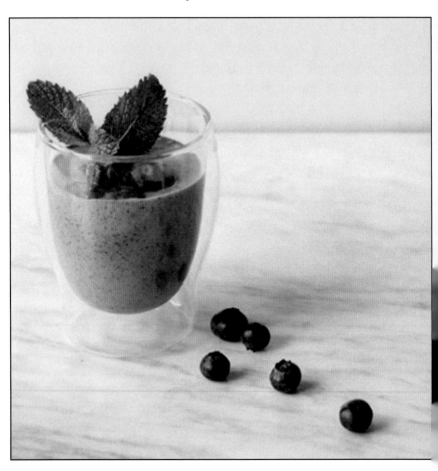

Ready for something tasty yet beautiful? Throw it all in a blender and admire the deep purple hue. Its tartness from the blueberries followed by a minty flourish might make you forget you're eating healthy now.

Prep Time: 5 min, Serve: 1

Ingredients

- 1 cup spinach
- 1 cup blueberry
- 1/2 kiwi
- 2 large mint leaves
- 1/2 cup coconut water
- 1/2 cup ice

Directions

Put all ingredients in a blender and mix it up until smooth.

Why This is Good For You

- High in vitamin A
- Very high in vitamin B6
- High in vitamin C
- High in vitamin E

Nutrition Facts

Calories 398, Calories from Fat 164, Total Fat 18.2g, Saturated Fat 12.1g, Trans Fat 0.0g, Sodium 215mg, Potassium 999mg, Total Carbohydrates 60.1g, Dietary Fiber 7.0g, Sugars 38.9g, Protein 5.3g.

4. Spiral of Flax and Oats Smoothie

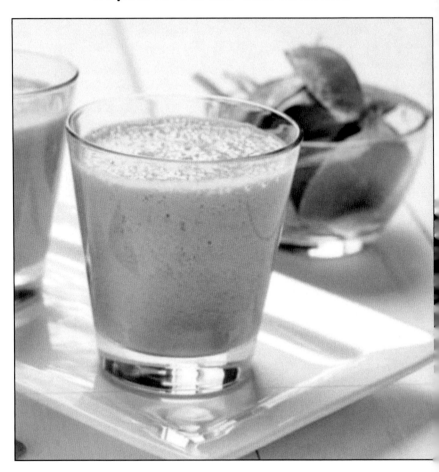

Have you ever been craving a slice of dessert bread, but really know you should have a smoothie instead? This one is for you. Banana, oats, milk and flax keep this treat true to the theme along with plenty of spinach. Don't forget to add a spiral of flax in the glass with an extra drizzle of milk.

Prep Time: 5 min, Serve: 2

Ingredients

- 1 banana
- 1-1/2 cup milk
- 4 big handfuls spinach
- 1/2 cup raw rolled oats
- 1 scoop Vega Choc-a-Lot (or similar)
- 2 tablespoons flax
- Ancient Granola topping

Directions

Put all ingredients except topping into a blender blend until smooth. Serve with topping.

Why This is Good For You

- Low in cholesterol
- Low in sodium
- High in calcium
- High in dietary fiber
- High in manganese
- High in vitamin C

Nutrition Facts

Calories 241, Calories from Fat 63, Total Fat 7.0g, Saturated Fat 2.0g, Trans Fat 0.0g, Cholesterol 12mg, Sodium 109mg, Potassium 315mg, Total Carbohydrates 35.1g, Dietary Fiber 7.5g, Sugars 15.0g, Protein 11.5g.

5. Sweet Honeydew Sensation

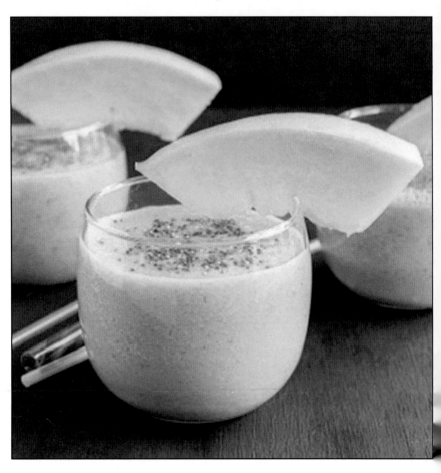

Expand your boundaries with this fresh and bold concoction. Honeydew, coconut milk, mint and lime juice combine into a wonderfully rich and delicious flavor. Enhance it further with a little honey or coconut nectar. This one takes a little extra time, but proves itself worth the effort. You'll know why it's called "Sensation" with your very first taste.

Prep Time: 10 min, Serve: 2

Ingredients

- 1/4 honeydew melon, cut into chunks
- 1/4 cup light coconut milk
- 1-2 leaves fresh mint (plus more for garnish)
- 1/4 teaspoon fresh lime juice (or to taste)
- 1 cup ice
- Drizzle of honey or coconut nectar, to taste

Directions

Cut melon in half, remove the seeds, and slice away the outer rind. Cut the melon into chunks, and add to your blender along with the coconut milk, mint, lime, and ice. Blend until smooth. Taste, then adjust sweetness with honey or coconut nectar. Serve with a garnish of mint, or fresh melon slices.

Why This is Good For You

- Low in cholesterol
- High in calcium
- High in phosphorus
- High in potassium
- Very high in vitamin C

Nutrition Facts

Calories 177, Calories from Fat 9, Total Fat 1.0g, Saturated Fat 0.5g, Trans Fat 0.0g, Cholesterol 3mg, Sodium 52mg, Potassium 359mg, Total Carbohydrates 14.1g, Dietary Fiber 0.7g, Sugars 12.9g, Protein 3.6g.

6. Piña Avocado Shiver

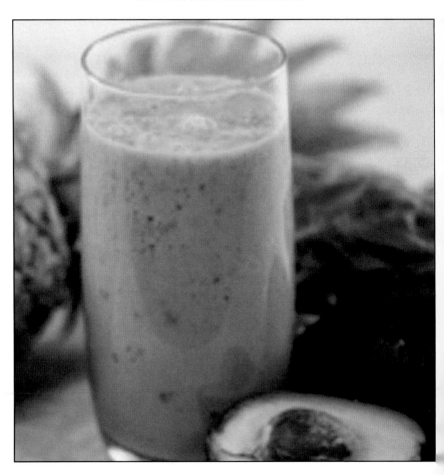

Something smooth, sweet and just a little tart. Perfect for a warm afternoon.Pineapple and avocado bring a hint of sweetness to the richness of almond milk and protein powder, intertwining with kale into one hearty beverage. If you're craving a shake, this one will send shivers down your spine.

Prep Time: 10 min, Serve: 1

Ingredients

- 1/3 cup unsweetened vanilla almond milk
- 1 large handful kale
- 1/6 cup pineapple chunks ➢ 1/4 ripe avocado
- 1/2 scoop protein powder (optional)
- 1 cup ice cubes

Directions

Put all ingredients into a blender and puree until smooth.

Why This is Good For You

- No cholesterol
- Very low in sodium
- Very high in manganese
- Very high in vitamin A
- Very high in vitamin C

Nutrition Facts

Calories 434, Calories from Fat 347, Total Fat 38.6g, Saturated Fat 33.9g, Trans Fat 0.0g, Cholesterol 0mg, Sodium 60mg, Potassium 817mg, Total Carbohydrates 24.2g, Dietary Fiber 5.9g, Sugars 13.1g, Protein 6.1g.

7. Peachy King Smoothie

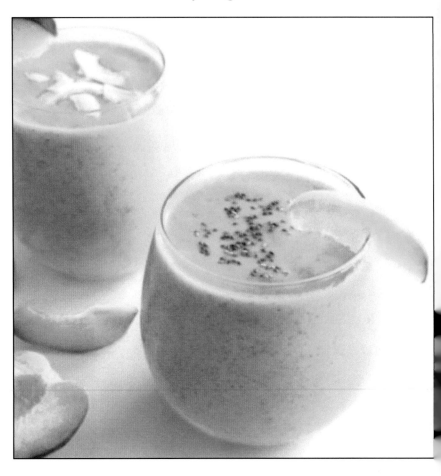

Pineapple, banana, vanilla and almond milk join with peaches to create one truly excellent blend. Fresh peaches create a summertime delight. You might call this one "peachy-keen"? Oh yeah, I went there.

Prep Time: 10 min, Serve: 2

Ingredients

- 4 scoops Daily Burn Fuel-6 in vanilla (optional)
- 2 cups unsweetened almond milk
- 2 cups frozen peaches
- 1 cup frozen pineapple
- 1 banana
- 4 cups kale
- 2 tablespoons ground flaxseed

Directions

Add all ingredients to blender. Mix until smooth.

Why This is Good For You

- Low in saturated fat
- No cholesterol
- Low in sodium
- High in dietary fiber
- High in manganese
- High in potassium
- Very high in vitamin A
- Very high in vitamin C

Nutrition Facts

Calories 124, Calories from Fat 17, Total Fat 1.9g, Saturated Fat 0.2g, Trans Fat 0.0g, Cholesterol 0mg, Sodium 60mg, Potassium 489mg, Total Carbohydrates 25.1g, Dietary Fiber 4.1g, Sugars 19.2g, Protein 4.4g.

8. Ginger Curve Smoothie

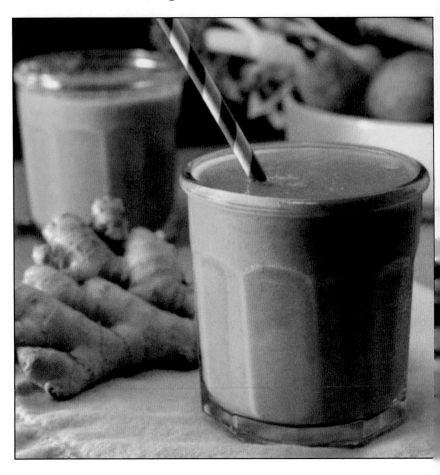

A light smoothie composed of navel orange, banana, ginger and some leafy greens. This fiber-rich blend is a perfect drink to get you going on a long day, especially one at the office. Try labeling your cup "wasabi" as a joke and coworkers will never look at you the same way again.

Prep Time: 8 min, Serve: 1

Ingredients

- 3/4 cups filtered water
- 2 generous handfuls fresh spinach
- 2 romaine leaves (optional)
- 1 navel orange
- 1 ripe banana
- 1" knob of fresh ginger (to taste), peel off skin with a spoon
- 1/2 cucumber (optional) peel if not organic

Directions

Rinse and prep veggies. If you have a high-powered blender, throw everything in and blend until smooth. If not, first blend the spinach and romaine until smooth, then add the remaining ingredients and blend. Pour into a glass and enjoy!

Why This is Good For You

- Low in saturated fat
- Very low in cholesterol
- Low in sodium
- Very high in manganese
- High in potassium
- Very high in vitamin A
- Very high in vitamin C

Nutrition Facts

Calories 183, Calories from Fat 15, Total Fat 1.7g, Saturated Fat 0.7g, Trans Fat 0.0g, Cholesterol 3mg, Sodium 60mg, Potassium 727mg, Total Carbohydrates 25.7g, Dietary Fiber 3.8g, Sugars 26.7g, Protein 5.9g.

9. Green Creator Smoothie

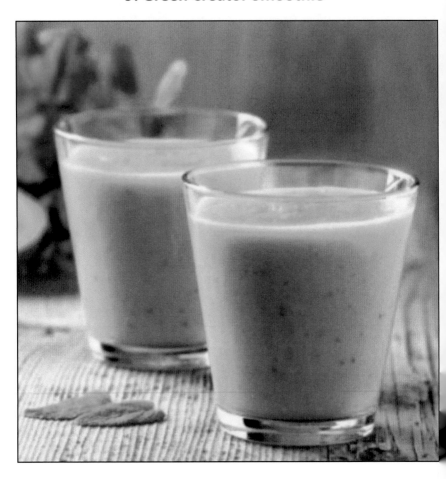

Sweet and smooth, but just unique enough to feel creative. Swiss chard and spirulina powder add a whole new dimension to this banana, avocado and kiwi treat. Making it is easier than it looks.

Prep Time: 5 min, Serve: 2

Ingredients

- 2 kiwis
- 1/2 avocado
- 2 Swiss chard leaves
- 2 bananas
- 4 tablespoons hemp seeds
- 2 teaspoons spirulina powder
- 2 cups coconut water
- 2 large handful of ice

Directions

Add all ingredients to blender and blend until smooth.

Why This is Good For You

- No saturated fat
- No cholesterol
- Very low in sodium
- High in iron
- Very high in vitamin B6
- Very high in vitamin B12
- Very high in vitamin C

Nutrition Facts

Calories 185, Calories from Fat 5, Total Fat 0.5g, Saturated Fat 0.1g, Trans Fat 0.0g, Sodium 55mg, Potassium 915mg, Total Carbohydrates 46.4g, Dietary Fiber 9.6g, Sugars 27.9g, Protein 3.4g.

10. Super Green Mango

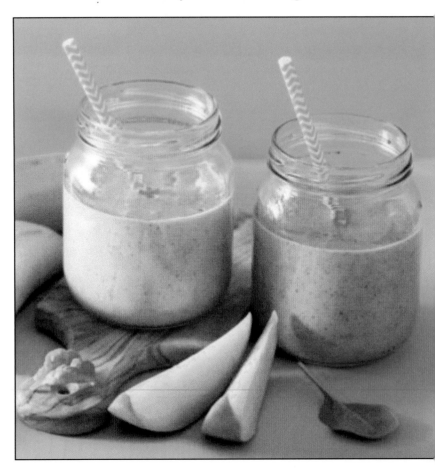

Tangy orange juice blends with the sweetness of bananas and mango in a base of coconut milk. The vitamins packed in this smoothie are a great way to really give yourself a hand in the afternoon. Its flavor is reminiscent of a fresh mango lasse from the finest Indian restaurant. Not just Green. Super Green.

Prep Time: 5 min, Serve: 4

Ingredients

- Handful of fresh spinach
- 2 frozen bananas. If using fresh bananas, then add a few ice cubes.
- 4 cups lite coconut milk
- 1/2 cup frozen mango chunks
- 1/2 cup orange juice
- 4 tablespoons hemp seeds

Directions

Mix All ingredients in a mixer mix well until smooth. Your delicious smoothie is now ready to serve.

Why This is Good For You

- Very low in saturated fat
- No cholesterol
- Very low in sodium
- High in dietary fiber
- Very high in vitamin A
- Very high in vitamin C

Nutrition Facts

Calories 190, Calories from Fat 0, Total Fat 0g, Saturated Fat 0g, Cholesterol 0mg, Sodium 10mg, Carbohydrates 48g, Dietary Fiber 0g, Sugars 43g, Protein 0g.

11. Pomegranate Orange Punch

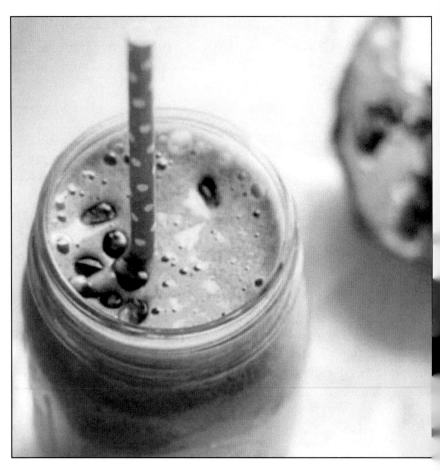

Light, sweet and goes down easy. Even with four bananas, oranges and cups of spinach, it's really the pomegranate that makes this smoothie wonderful. But careful with the pomegranate seeds! They burst easily and spray really far when they do. You don't want to go to work with a purple streak across your face. Call it wisdom born of experience.

Prep Time: 5 min, Serve: 4

Ingredients

- 4 cups spinach, fresh
- 2 cups water
- 4 oranges, peeled
- 2 cups pomegranate seeds
- 4 bananas

Directions

Blend spinach and water until smooth. Next add the fruits and blend again. Save a few pomegranates for a sprinkle.

Why This is Good For You

- No saturated fat
- No cholesterol
- Very low in sodium
- High in dietary fiber
- Very high in vitamin C

Nutrition Facts

Calories 370, Calories from Fat 17, Total Fat 1.9g, Saturated Fat 0g, Cholesterol 0mg, Sodium 0mg, Carbohydrates 63g, Dietary Fiber 4g, Sugars 0g, Protein 20g.

12. Cilantro Limeade

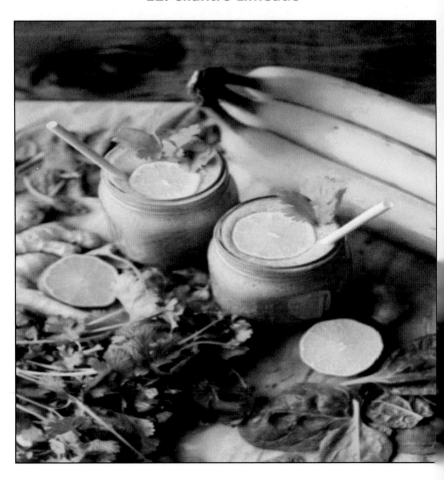

Sweet fruity taste with just a little bite. Limes, cilantro and ginger are certainly a bold choice in conjunction with spinach and bananas. If you have ever dreamed of eating spiced fruit, then look no farther than Cilantro Limeade. This one really walks on the wild side.

Prep Time: 5 min, Serve: 4

Ingredients

- 3 cups spinach, fresh
- 1 cup cilantro, fresh
- 4 cups water
- 6 bananas
- 2 limes
- 2 inches fresh ginger (add slowly and adjust to taste)

Directions

Blend spinach, ginger, cilantro and water until smooth. Next, add the remaining fruits and blend again.

Why This is Good For You

- Very low in saturated fat
- Very low in sodium
- High in dietary fiber
- High in manganese
- High in potassium
- High in vitamin A
- Very high in vitamin B6
- Very high in vitamin C

Nutrition Facts

Calories 146, Calories from Fat 1, Total Fat 0.1g, Saturated Fat 0.1g, Trans Fat 0.0g, Sodium 10mg, Potassium 638mg, Total Carbohydrates 37.1g, Dietary Fiber 4.9g, Sugars 18.5g, Protein 1.9g.

13. Avocado Dream

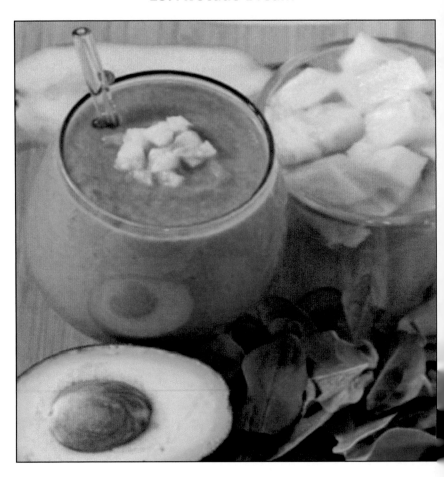

A dream without ice cream. You can tell your friends about it, but they may not believe it was real. Pineapple, avocado, spinach, bananas and your choice of base. All these meaty fruits make the Avocado Dream almost creamy.

Prep Time: 5 min, Serve: 4

Ingredients

- 1 cup pineapple chunks
- 1 avocado, diced
- 2 cup fresh spinach
- 1/2 cup pineapple juice (almond milk, soy milk or any other liquid will work)
- 2 tablespoons flaxseed (optional)
- 2 bananas (cut into slices)

Directions

In a blender, process pineapple, avocado, spinach, juice, flaxseed and frozen banana until smooth. Serve chilled.

Why This is Good For You

- No cholesterol
- Very low in sodium
- High in dietary fiber
- High in manganese
- High in vitamin C

Nutrition Facts

Calories 273, Calories from Fat, 134 Total Fat, 14.9g, Saturated Fat 2.1g, Trans Fat 0.0g, Cholesterol 0mg, Sodium 11mg, Potassium 763mg, Total Carbohydrates 35.8g, Dietary Fiber 7.1g, Sugars 21.7g, Protein 2.7g

14. Strawberry Peach Refresher

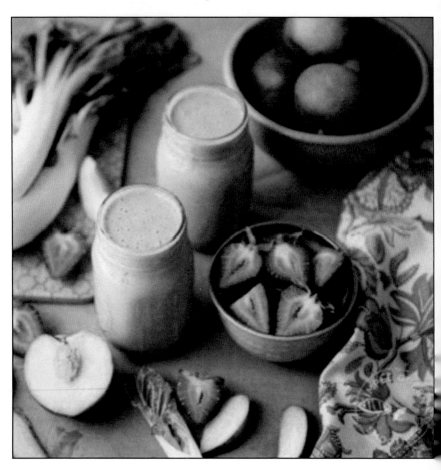

Surprise your friends with this secret ingredient. Bok Choy is a common leafy green in Asian cuisine, but not so much for Americans. Add peaches and some strawberries, and you get this deceptively creamy treat for so few calories, compliments of the almond milk. This smoothie with its secret ingredient will be quite the conversation piece.

Prep Time: 5 min, Serve: 1

Ingredients

- 1 cup bok choy, fresh
- 1 cup almond milk, unsweetened
- 1/2 cup strawberries
- 1 cup peaches

Directions

Blend bok choy and almond milk until smooth. Next add the remaining fruits and blend again.

Why This is Good For You

- No saturated fat
- No cholesterol
- No sodium
- High in dietary fiber
- Very high in vitamin C

Nutrition Facts

Calories 90, Calories from Fat 0, Total Fat 0g, Saturated Fat 0g, Polyunsaturated Fat 0g, Monounsaturated Fat 0g, Cholesterol 0mg, Sodium 0mg, Potassium 0mg, Carbohydrates 7g, Dietary Fiber 4g, Sugars 20g, Protein 0g.

15. Shamrock Shake

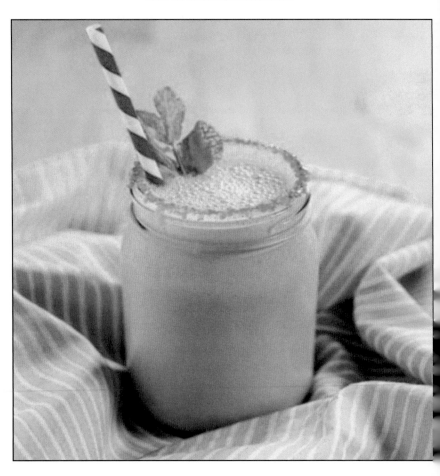

The milk, mint, yogurt and vanilla combine with kale and banana to forge a healthy alternative to an otherwise authentic Shamrock Shake. Everything about it practically sings "Top of the morning to you" while it gives the rest of the day to you, as well.

Prep Time: 5 min, Serve: 1

Ingredients

- 1/2 cup milk (I used Almond Milk, but you can use any milk you choose)
- 1/2 cup plain Greek yogurt
- 1/4 cup kale
- 1/4 teaspoon vanilla extract
- 1/8 teaspoon mint extract or about 2 drops Peppermint Essential Oil

Directions

Put all ingredients into a blender, and blend until smooth. Pour into a glass to serve.

Why This is Good For You

- Very high in calcium
- High in iron
- High in manganese
- High in magnesium
- High in phosphorus
- High in potassium
- High in riboflavin
- Very high in vitamin A
- High in vitamin C

Nutrition Facts

Calories 268, Calories from Fat 78, Total Fat 8.7g, Saturated Fat 2.5g, Trans Fat 0.0g, Sodium 265mg, Potassium 1223mg, Total Carbohydrates 30.6g, Dietary Fiber 5.6g, Sugars 20.8g, Protein 25.0g.

16. Vanilla Lime Twist Smoothie

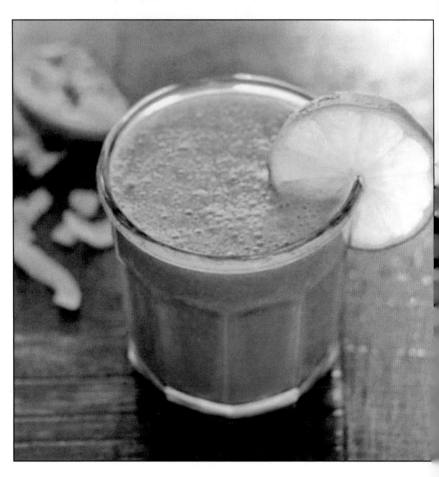

Vanilla yogurt, spinach, banana, lime juice, honey, milk and vanilla extract. Its myriad ingredients and creamy base are met by surprisingly few calories. Sweet with just a hint of tart and a smooth finish. This one almost begs to be taken by the pool, so why not? Show off that body you've been tuning up with all these smoothies.

Prep Time: 5 min, Serve: 2

Ingredients

- 1 cup vanilla yogurt
- 2 cups spinach leaves, packed
- 4 teaspoons honey
- 1 banana, best frozen
- 4 tablespoons fresh lime juice
- 1 teaspoon vanilla extract
- 1 cup milk
- 1 cup ice (optional)

Directions

Place all ingredients except the ice in a blender and puree until blended. Add ice and puree until smooth. Pour into a glass and serve with a straw.

Why This is Good For You

- Very low in saturated fat
- Low in cholesterol
- Very high in calcium
- High in manganese
- High in riboflavin
- Very high in vitamin A
- High in vitamin B12
- Very high in vitamin C
- High in vitamin E

Nutrition Facts

Calories 164, Calories from Fat 13, Total Fat 1.4g, Saturated Fat 0.1g, Trans Fat 0.0g, Cholesterol 5mg, Sodium 148mg, Potassium 564mg, Total Carbohydrates 25.1g, Dietary Fiber 3.6g Sugars 11.8g, Protein 14.1g.

17. Spinach Magic

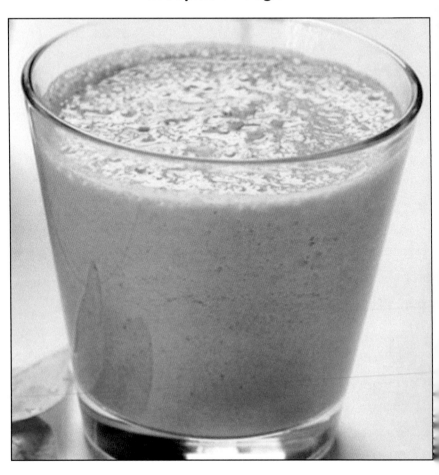

A magical concoction of spinach, honey, almond milk, Greek yogurt, peanut butter and chocolate protein powder; this smoothie is thick, rich and full of essential nutrients. It's simple to make because all the ingredients are either half a tablespoon or one cup. Just scoop, drop and hit the button. Then tap the blender 3 times with a chop stick and yell delectamentum! That's where the magic comes in.

Prep Time: 5 min, Serve: 2

Ingredients

- 1/2 tablespoon honey
- 1 cup Spinach
- 1 cup Vanilla Almond Milk
- 1/2 cup plain Greek yogurt
- 1/2 tablespoon Peanut Butter
- 1/2 tablespoon Chocolate Protein Powder (optional)
- 1/2 tablespoon Chia Seeds

Directions

Blend everything together. Serve with a straw.

Why This is Good For You

- Low in cholesterol
- High in calcium
- High in manganese
- High in phosphorus
- High in potassium
- High in riboflavin
- Very high in vitamin A
- High in vitamin B6
- Very high in vitamin C

Nutrition Facts

Calories 195, Calories from Fat 23, Total Fat 2.6g, Saturated Fat 1.4g, Trans Fat 0.0g, Cholesterol 7mg, Sodium 111mg, Potassium 802mg, Total Carbohydrates 37.8g, Dietary Fiber 4.6g, Sugars 26.8g, Protein 8.9g.

18. Power of Green Tea

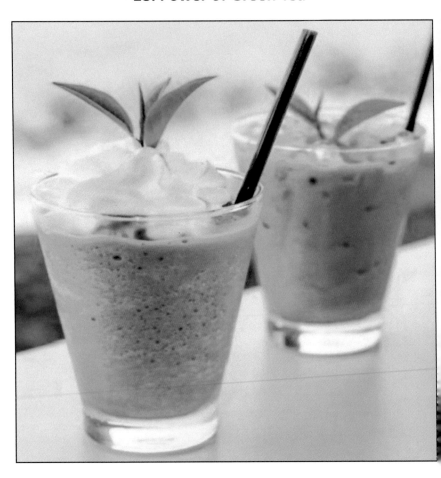

Antioxidant-rich green tea makes this healthy smoothie a nutritional powerhouse. Throw in baby spinach, banana and grapes to really bring out the power. Garnish it with whipped cream on top, briefly marvel at its majestic beauty, then enjoy as a summertime treat!

Prep Time: 5 min, Serve: 2

Ingredients

- 3/4 cup green grapes
- 1/2 cup baby spinach
- 1/2 cup frozen banana slices
- 1/2 cup green tea (liquid)

Directions

Put all ingredients in a blender and blend until smooth.

Why This is Good For You

- Very low in sodium
- Very high in vitamin A
- High in vitamin C

Nutrition Facts

Calories 314, Calories from Fat 0, Total Fat 0g, Sodium 55mg, Carbohydrates 76g, Dietary Fiber 2g, Sugars 71g, Protein 1g.

19. Kiwi Fantasy

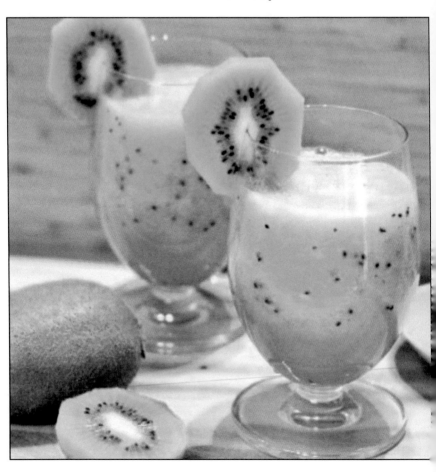

Take a step into fantasy with this fruit-packed smoothie recipe. Kiwi, spinach, banana, vanilla yogurt, flax seed and some apple juice for that little extra twist. You can never go wrong with kiwi. The end result will be a light shake almost like Italian Ice, making this smoothie the ideal companion for a nice warm day of sunbathing.

Prep Time: 5 min, Serve: 1

Ingredients

- 1 kiwi, peeled and halved
- 1/4 banana, peeled
- 1/2 cup baby spinach
- 1/4 cup vanilla yogurt
- 1 tablespoon ground flax seed (optional)
- 1/4 cup apple juice
- 5-6 ice cubes

Directions

Place all the ingredients into a blender. Blend until smooth. Garnish with a kiwi slice.

Why This is Good For You

- Low in saturated fat
- No cholesterol
- High in dietary fiber
- Very high in manganese
- High in magnesium
- High in potassium
- Very high in vitamin
- A Very high in vitamin C

Nutrition Facts

Calories 146, Calories from Fat 59, Total Fat 6.6g, Saturated Fat 0.6g, Trans Fat 0.0g, Cholesterol 0mg, Sodium 89mg, Potassium 648mg, Total Carbohydrates 20.3g, Dietary Fiber 5.2g, Sugars 11.9g, Protein 4.7g.

20. Cranberry Kickstart

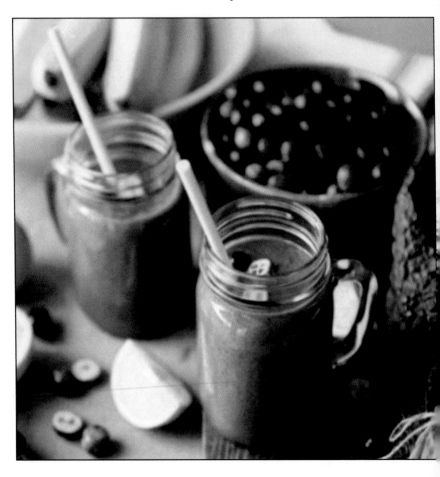

Kale, cranberries, an orange and a banana—a Vitamin C booster! This smoothie is remarkable for being light and for its rich brown color. Slurp down this smoothie at breakfast to kick your day into high gear and keep you satisfied until lunchtime. The kale means it's loaded with minerals, making it ideal for days you expect to sweat.

Prep Time: 5 min, Serve: 1

Ingredients

- 1 cup fresh kale
- 1/2 cup water
- 1/2 cup cranberries
- 1 orange, peeled
- 1 banana

Directions

Blend kale and water until smooth. Next add the remaining fruits and blend again.

Why This is Good For You

- Low in saturated fat
- Low in sodium
- High in dietary fiber
- High in vitamin B12
- High in vitamin C

Nutrition Facts

Calories 310, Calories from Fat 30, Total Fat 3.3g, Saturated Fat 0.5g, Trans Fat 0.0g, Sodium 69mg, Potassium 617mg, Total Carbohydrates 77.4g, Dietary Fiber 9.0g, Sugars 38.1g, Protein 4.4g.

21. Mango-Coconut Duster

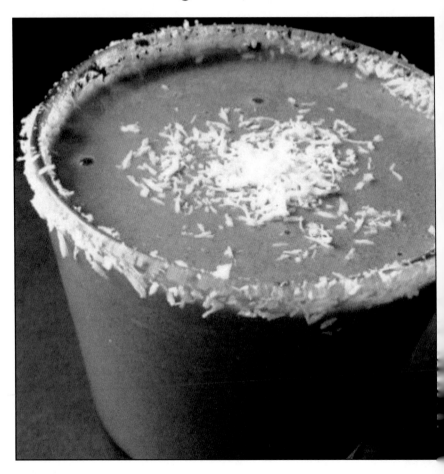

Stricken by the mood for a snack both functional and stylish? Then grab some spinach, mango cubes, a bit of banana, coconut milk and orange juice. Don't forget to check out the optional ingredients. Dust it with coconut shavings for the added flair. This decadently thick smoothie recipe can keep your hunger sated for hours.

Prep Time: 5 min, Serve: 1

Ingredients

- 1/2 cup fresh washed spinach leaves, packed
- 1/2 cup fresh or frozen mango cubes
- 1/4 medium banana
- 3/8 cup light coconut milk
- 1/4 cup orange juice
- 1/4 cup ice cubes OPTIONAL ADDITIONS:
- 1/2 tablespoon coconut butter
- 1/2 tablespoon ground flaxseeds
- Chopped mango or coconut for topping

Directions

Place all ingredients in a blender and puree until smooth. Pour into glasses, add toppings if desired, and serve with a straw.

Why This is Good For You

- No cholesterol
- Very low in sodium
- Very high in vitamin C

Nutrition Facts

Calories 295, Calories from Fat 69, Total Fat 7.7g, Saturated Fat 6.5g, Trans Fat 0.0g, Cholesterol 0mg, Sodium 17mg, Potassium 569mg, Total Carbohydrates 59.2g, Dietary Fiber 3.0g, Sugars 53.6g, Protein 1.4g.

22. Christmas Morning Bliss

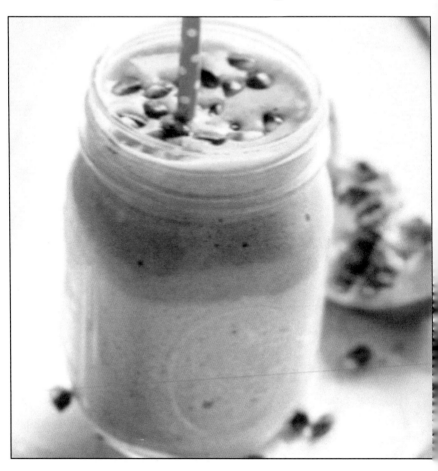

Remember what it was like to wake up as a child on Christmas morning? This two-layer technique creates a red and green color combination that will bliss you back into those fond childhood memories. Sprinkle some crushed peppermints on top to enhance the experience. Consider starting a new family tradition by serving this delicious smoothie to your family on Christmas morning.

Prep Time: 5 min, Serve: 2

Ingredients (pink layer)

- 2 frozen bananas
- 2 cups frozen strawberries (or fresh!)
- 1cup coconut water

Ingredients (green layer)

- 2 cups fresh spinach
- 1 frozen banana
- 1/2 cup pomegranate arils
- 1/2 cup coconut water

Directions

First, prepare pink layer add all ingredients in a blender blend until smooth. Then pour into half portion of glass. Add all green layer ingredients in a blender and blend until smooth. Pour into the remaining part of glass.

Why This is Good For You

- Very low in saturated fat
- Very low in sodium
- High in dietary fiber
- Very high in manganese
- High in potassium
- Very high in vitamin C

Nutrition Facts

Calories 176, Calories from Fat 9, Total Fat 1.0g, Saturated Fat 0.1g, Trans Fat 0.0g, Sodium 14mg, Potassium 781mg, Total Carbohydrates 42.1g, Dietary Fiber 6.1g, Sugars 31.1g, Protein 2.1g.

23. Amazing Apricot

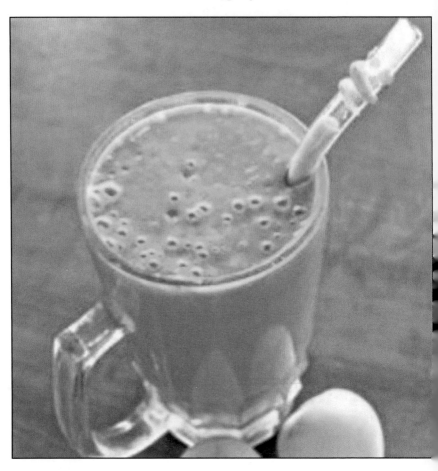

Apricots are a hit-or-miss sort of fruit. Sometimes they can be super sweet, and other times, they can rather blah. Using them in a smoothie is a great alternative to get the distinctive apricot-y-ness without the flavor disappointment. This recipe uses local honey to elevate the flavor profile.

Prep Time: 5 min, Serve: 1

Ingredients

- 1 cup water
- 1/2 cup apricots
- drizzle of local honey
- 1/2 banana
- 1/2 cup romaine lettuce (or spinach)

Directions

Blend all the ingredients together until smooth.

Why This is Good For You

- Low in saturated fat
- Low in cholesterol
- Very high in calcium
- High in manganese
- High in potassium
- High in vitamin A
- Very high in vitamin C

Nutrition Facts

Calories 181, Calories from Fat 13, Total Fat 1.5g, Saturated Fat 0.6g, Trans Fat 0.0g, Cholesterol 9mg, Sodium 170mg, Potassium 864mg, Total Carbohydrates 32.3g, Dietary Fiber 3.6g, Sugars 26.6g, Protein 12.7g.

24. Crazy Coconut

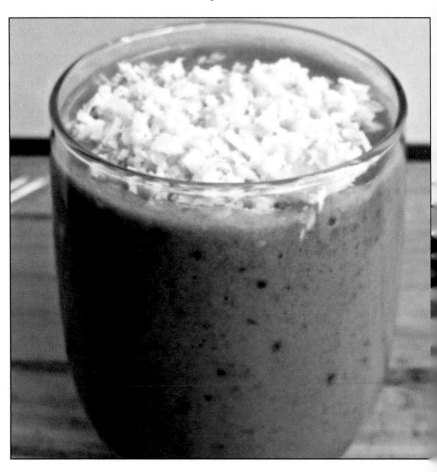

Coconut, pineapple and spinach. Thick like a milkshake, this coconut-infused smoothie recipe transports you to a tropical island. And then leaves you there. Nice job, Magellan.

Prep Time: 5 min, Serve: 1

Ingredients

- 1/2 cup water
- 1/2 pineapple
- 1/4 cup coconut flakes, more to garnish
- 1/2 cup spinach

Directions

Put all ingredients together in a blender and blend until smooth.

Why This is Good For You

- No cholesterol
- High in dietary fiber
- Very high in manganese
- High in potassium
- High in vitamin A
- High in vitamin B6
- Very high in vitamin C

Nutrition Facts

Calories 353, Calories from Fat 95, Total Fat 10.6g, Saturated Fat 2.3g, Trans Fat 0.0g, Cholesterol 0mg, Sodium 273mg, Potassium 1453mg, Total Carbohydrates 54.3g, Dietary Fiber 9.5g, Sugars 44.9g, Protein 4.1g.

25. Frugal

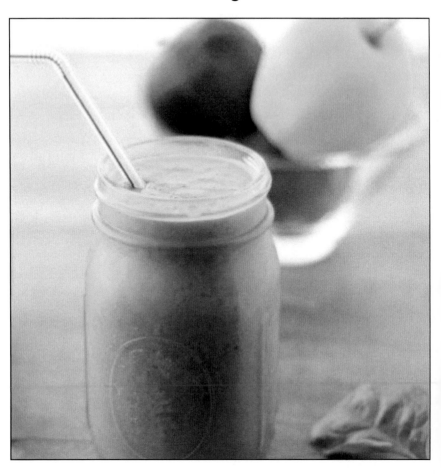

Start your day with this energetic smoothie that's packed with what your body needs but is budget friendly. It earns its name by ingredients even the tightest penny-pincher would have in the pantry: apple, banana and cucumber.

Prep Time: 5 min, Serve: 1

Ingredients

- 1/2 cup water
- 1 sweet apple (like Red Delicious or Gala)
- 1/2 banana
- 1/4 cucumber

Directions

Blend all the ingredients together until smooth.

Why This is Good For You

- Very low in saturated fat
- No cholesterol
- Very high in calcium
- High in dietary fiber
- Very high in manganese
- High in potassium
- Very high in vitamin A
- Very high in vitamin C
- High in vitamin E

Nutrition Facts

Calories 290, Calories from Fat 49, Total Fat 5.4g, Saturated Fat 0.2g, Trans Fat 0.0g, Cholesterol 0mg, Sodium 240mg, Potassium 1290mg, Total Carbohydrates 68.1g, Dietary Fiber 12.6g, Sugars 40.0g, Protein 7.8g.

26. Citrus Cooler

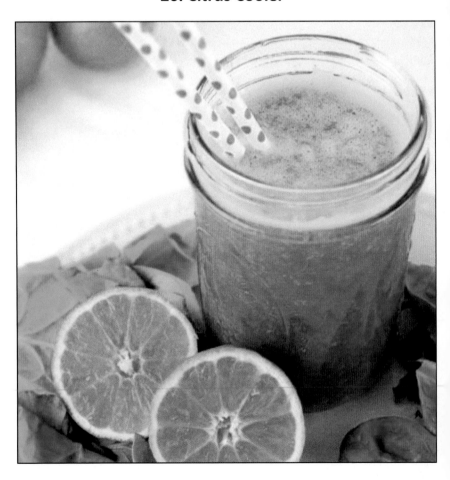

A delectably tart blend of oranges, pineapple and spinach. Simple and crisp, this smoothie carries a ton of nutrition in a light, refreshing blend. Wow your friends by serving this on a Sunday morning brunch.

Prep Time: 5 min, Serve: 4

Ingredients

- 2 cups water
- 2 cups pineapple
- 2 oranges
- 2 cups spinach

Directions

Put all ingredients together in a blender and blend until smooth.

Why This is Good For You

- Very low in saturated fat
- No cholesterol
- Very low in sodium
- High in manganese
- High in vitamin A
- Very high in vitamin C

Nutrition Facts

Calories 346, Calories from Fat 5, Total Fat 0.6g, Saturated Fat 0.1g, Trans Fat 0.0g, Cholesterol 0mg, Sodium 49mg, Potassium 825mg, Total Carbohydrates 84.9g, Dietary Fiber 7.6g, Sugars 68.2g, Protein 3.5g.

27. Raspberry Ripple

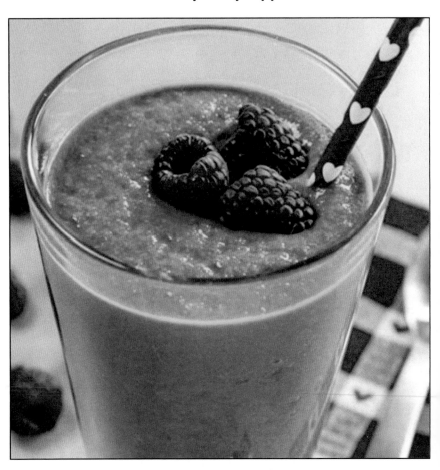

Pak choi is often mislabeled baby bok choi, so don't panic. Pak choi is easily found in most grocery stores these days. It is a great way to add green variety to your smoothies if you're tired of spinach. Playfully add a banana with a ripple of raspberries throughout. Double up on the ripples by dropping a few extra raspberries into the glass.

Prep Time: 5 min, Serve : 1

Ingredients

- 1 cup water
- 1/2 cup raspberries
- 1/2 banana
- 1/2 cup pak choi (aka, baby bok choi)

Directions

Put all ingredients together in a blender; blend until smooth.

Why This is Good For You

- Low in saturated fat
- No cholesterol
- Very low in sodium
- High in dietary fiber
- High in manganese
- High in magnesium
- Very high in vitamin C

Nutrition Facts

Calories 348, Calories from Fat 93, Total Fat 10.3g, Saturated Fat 1.0g, Trans Fat 0.0g, Cholesterol 0mg, Sodium 41mg, Potassium 1035mg, Total Carbohydrates 57.1g, Dietary Fiber 17.5g, Sugars 21.2g, Protein 14.2g.

28. Island Blast

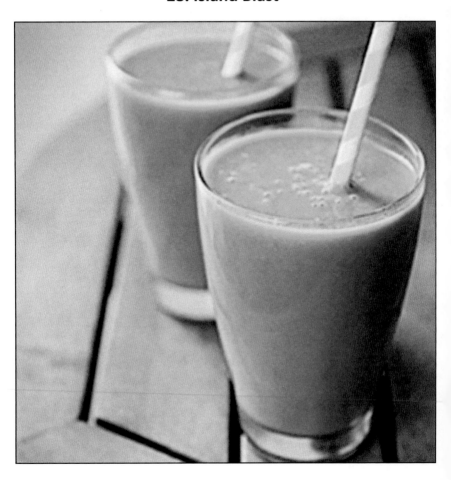

Are you in the mood for a smoothie so flavorful that it sends your mind on an island getaway? Then try this mix of banana, pineapple, ginger, parsley, ginger, celery and cucumber. Chock-full of necessary nutrients, this smoothie tastes like a vacation in a glass. Don't forget to fire your travel agent.

Prep Time: 5 min Serve: 1

Ingredients

- 1/2 small banana (ripe and peeled)
- 1/2 rib of celery
- 1/8 cucumber
- 1/2 cup of fresh or frozen pineapple
- 1/2 small handful of parsley
- 1/4 inch piece of ginger
- 1 cup of coconut water

Directions

Blend all the ingredients together until smooth.

Why This is Good For You

- Low in sodium
- High in niacin
- Very high in vitamin C

Nutrition Facts

Calories 170, Calories from Fat 0, Total Fat 0g, Sodium 50mg, Potassium 130mg, Carbohydrates 42g, Sugars 42g, Protein 0g.

29. Minty Papaya Magic

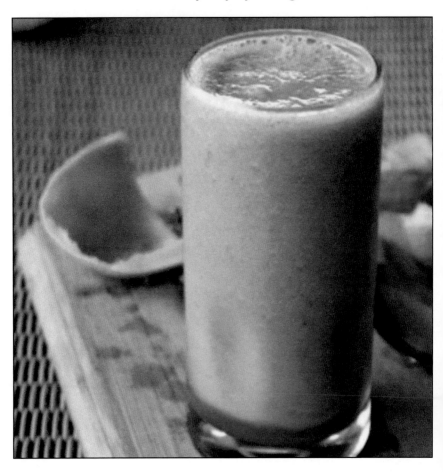

Now for a bit of the exotic. This is a novel blend of papaya, pear, goji berries, spinach and mint. The "magic" comes from the high levels of antioxidants entwined with a robust yet hauntingly familiar flavor. If you're not sure what a goji berry is, it's also called a wolfberry. They grow easily in my state of New Mexico. Try not to eat them all before they make it into the blender!

Prep Time: 5 min, Serve: 4

Ingredients

- 6 cups spinach leaves
- 4 cups cubed ripe papaya
- 2 cups cubed pear
- 4 tablespoons goji berries (dried or fresh)
- 20 fresh leaves of mint
- 2 cups filtered water

Directions

Pour water into blender. Add papaya first, followed by the pear, berries and then mint leaves. Add the spinach last.

Why This is Good For You

- Very low in cholesterol
- Very low in sodium
- High in dietary fiber
- Very high in manganese
- Very high in vitamin C

Nutrition Facts

Calories 218, Calories from Fat 42, Total Fat 4.7g, Saturated Fat 1.7g, Trans Fat 0.0g, Cholesterol 4mg, Sodium 33mg, Potassium 368mg, Total Carbohydrates 37.9g, Dietary Fiber 6.1g, Sugars 25.3g, Protein 9.6g.

30. Spinach and Collard Greens Smoothie

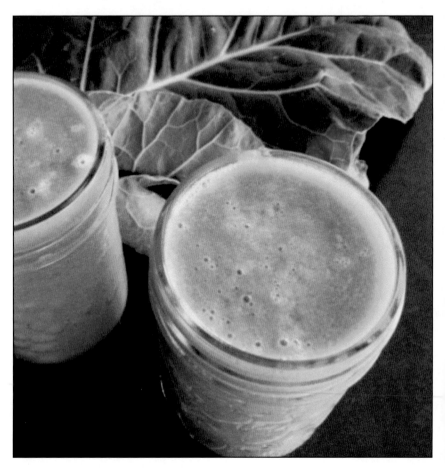

If you're from the American South, your mother probably tried for years to get you to eat collard greens. Who knew that today you would be doing it with a smile on your face? Loaded with vitamins, this one is a perfect way to scratch your grab-and-go (spin)itch. This green treat is made from spinach, collard greens, pineapple chunks and a bunch of oranges.

Prep Time: 10 min, Serve: 4

Ingredients

- 2 cups fresh spinach
- 2 cups fresh collard greens
- 8 whole medium sized oranges
- 6 cups pineapple chunks
- additional orange juice if needed to adjust thickness

Directions

Squeeze out the juice from the oranges. Use this fresh juice as a liquid base for blending the spinach and collard greens together. Blend at slow speed until smooth. Add the pineapples to the orange and greens mixture and blend at high speed until well mixed. Pour and serve immediately.

Why This is Good For You

- No saturated fat
- No cholesterol
- Low in sodium
- Very high in vitamin A
- Very high in vitamin C

Nutrition Facts

Calories 250, Calories from Fat 4, Total Fat 0.4g, Saturated Fat 0g, Polyunsaturated Fat 0g, Monounsaturated Fat 0g, Cholesterol 0mg, Sodium 82mg, Carbohydrates 60g, Dietary Fiber 4.3g, Sugars 53g, Protein 3g.

31. Zucchini Vanilla Tango

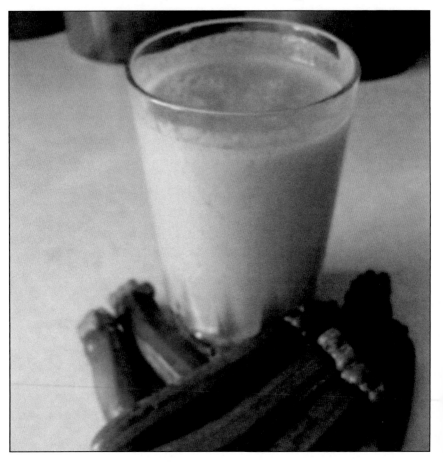

Can't give away the zucchini from your bumper garden crop this year? Your family threatening to disown you? Try this recipe to win back their favors. Nothing says "bold" like something lean, green, and "a little nutty." The vanilla and pinch of salt add just the flourish you need to make this smoothie dance memorable!

Prep Time: 5 min, Serve: 2

Ingredients

- 2 cups chopped zucchini
- 2 cups baby spinach
- 2 small bananas
- 4 tablespoons pecan nuts
- 4 tablespoons pitted dates
- 2 cups non-dairy milk (like soy or almond)
- 1 teaspoon pure vanilla extract
- A pinch of salt

Directions

Wash zucchini and spinach thoroughly. Without peeling, slice zucchini into half-inch thickness. Peel banana and cut into half-inch slices. Put zucchini, spinach, vanilla extract and milk in a blender and process until smooth. Add all the remaining ingredients and blend on high speed until smooth. Pour into a tall glass and serve with a sprinkle of crushed pecans.

Why This is Good For You

- Low in saturated fat
- Very high in calcium
- High in dietary fiber
- Very high in vitamin B6
- Very high in vitamin B12
- Very high in vitamin C
- High in vitamin E

Nutrition Facts

Calories 168, Calories from Fat 31, Total Fat 3.4g, Saturated Fat 0.3g, Trans Fat 0.0g, Cholesterol 14mg, Sodium 195mg, Potassium 457mg, Total Carbohydrates 22.0g, Dietary Fiber 4.4g, Sugars 14.7g, Protein 14.2g.

32. Sweet and Sour Green Smoothie

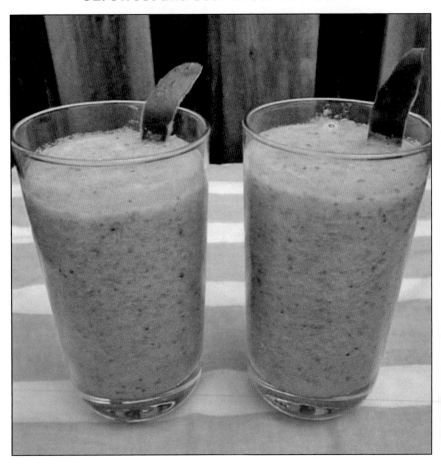

With grapefruit, apricots, dates and lots of superfood veggies, this smoothie stands apart from others in its creative blend of flavor. Save this one for the weekend when you can play around with the proportions to suit your taste buds. Marvel for a moment at its enchantingly marbled visage. Go boldly, do not be scared!

Prep Time: 5 min, Serve: 1

Ingredients

- 1/8 cup broccoli florets
- 1/8 cup cauliflower florets
- 1/4 pink grapefruit, peeled
- 1/4 tablespoon linseeds (optional)
- 1/4 tablespoon almond nuts
- 1 tablespoons dried pitted dates (pre-soaked for a smoother blend)
- 1/4 cup dried apricots
- 1/4 cup non-dairy milk
- 1 /2 cup water

Directions

Put water, milk, broccoli, cauliflower and grapefruit in a blender. Whiz until mixed thoroughly. Add linseeds, almonds, dates and apricots. Blend until smooth. Pour into a tall glass and enjoy.

Why This is Good For You

- No saturated fat
- No cholesterol
- Low in sodium
- Very high in manganese
- High in vitamin A
- High in vitamin B6
- High in vitamin B12
- Very high in vitamin C

Nutrition Facts

Calories 140, Calories from Fat, 0 Total Fat 0g, Saturated Fat 0g, Polyunsaturated Fat 0g, Monounsaturated Fat 0g, Cholesterol 0mg, Sodium 30mg, Potassium 420mg, Carbohydrates 33g, Dietary Fiber 2g, Sugars 30g, Protein 2g.

33. Green Muesli Smoothie

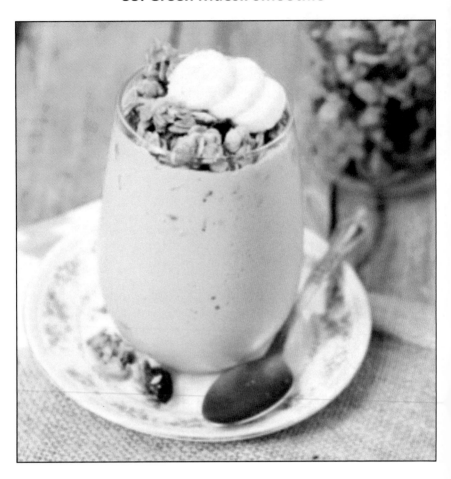

Put away your passport and try this international smoothie, straight from Switzerland. Muesli is akin to oatmeal with fruit, instead of milk. You may feel like you're Swiss while drinking this, but please resist the urge to wear skis in the kitchen.

Prep Time: 5 min, Serve: 2

Ingredients

- 1 cup ripe mango chunks
- 1 cup ripe bananas
- 1 cup muesli
- 2 tablespoons sesame seeds
- 1/2 cup pitted dates
- 1 cup non-dairy milk (like soy or almond)
- 1 cup distilled water

Directions

Place water, milk, muesli and lettuce in a blender. Mix thoroughly. Add remaining ingredients and continue blending until smooth. Pour into a tall glass and top with a little extra muesli and fruit.

Why This is Good For You

- Low in sodium
- High in dietary fiber
- High in manganese
- Very high in vitamin C

Nutrition Facts

Calories 348, Calories from Fat 177, Total Fat 19.7g, Saturated Fat 3.5g, Trans Fat 0.0g, Sodium 99mg, Potassium 723mg, Total Carbohydrates 61.3g, Dietary Fiber 15.7g, Sugars 23.7g, Protein 12.1g.

34. Strawberry and Oats Smoothie

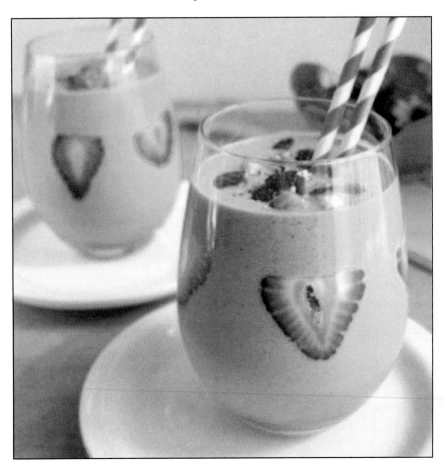

Packing fruit, milk and plenty of grains, this densely-nutritious blend is practically breakfast in a glass. Use a little bit of honey to stick slices of strawberries along the stemless wine glass glass prior to pouring in the smoothie to get an amazing presentation, but the true beauty of this smoothie is in its taste. This one would also be great for the Holiday season!

Prep Time: 5 min, Serve: 2

Ingredients

- 1 cup fresh strawberries
- 2 large stalks of celery
- 2 teaspoons Barley powder
- 1 cup instant oats
- 2 tablespoons pumpkin seeds
- 1 cup non-dairy milk (like soy or almond milk)
- drizzle of local honey (or agave nectar) to taste
- 1 cup distilled water
- 1 cup ice cubes

Directions

Cut celery into 2-inch strips so it becomes easier to process. Put celery, oats, ice cubes and water in a blender and whiz on high speed until smooth. Add strawberries, pumpkin seeds and milk and blend until smooth. Pour into a tall glass and serve with strawberry garnish.

Why This is Good For You

- Very low in saturated fat
- Very low in cholesterol
- Low in sodium
- High in calcium
- Very high in vitamin C

Nutrition Facts

Calories 316, Calories from Fat 16, Total Fat 1.8g, Saturated Fat 0.3g, Trans Fat 0.0g, Cholesterol 3mg, Sodium 91mg, Potassium 481mg, Total Carbohydrates 67.7g, Dietary Fiber 6.5g, Sugars 39.8g, Protein 11.5g.

35. Magic of Kale

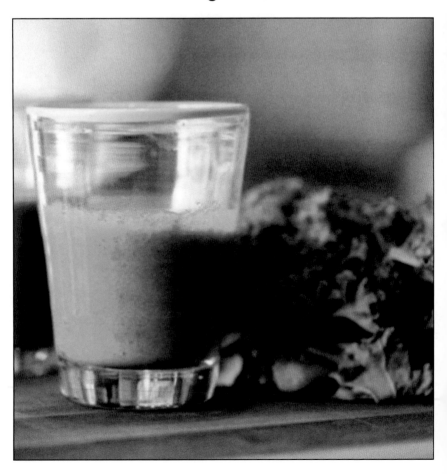

Wow! BAM! Zingers, Batman! This is a head-spinning blend of maple syrup, bananas, cashews and ginger. Smooth, sweet, nutty, and very robust. Once you taste it, you'll understand why it's magic. Save this one for your monthly Dungeons and Dragons game night.

Prep Time: 5 min, Serve: 1

Ingredients

- 1/2 cup green kale leaves
- 1 cup diced ripe bananas
- 1/4 cup raw cashew nuts
- 1/2 tablespoon maple syrup
- 1/2 teaspoon pure vanilla extract
- 1/4 teaspoon chopped ginger
- 1/2 cup filtered water
- 2 cups ice
- A pinch of salt to taste

Directions

Put all ingredients in a blender. Blend until smooth. Pour into glasses and serve.

Why This is Good For You

- No cholesterol
- Very low in sodium
- Very high in vitamin A
- Very high in vitamin C

Nutrition Facts

Calories 229, Calories from Fat 139, Total Fat 15.4g, Saturated Fat 1.2g, Trans Fat 0.0g, Cholesterol 0mg, Sodium 40mg, Potassium 437mg, Total Carbohydrates 23.2g, Dietary Fiber 3.0g, Sugars 11.6g, Protein 3.5g.

36. Caramel And Banana Butternut

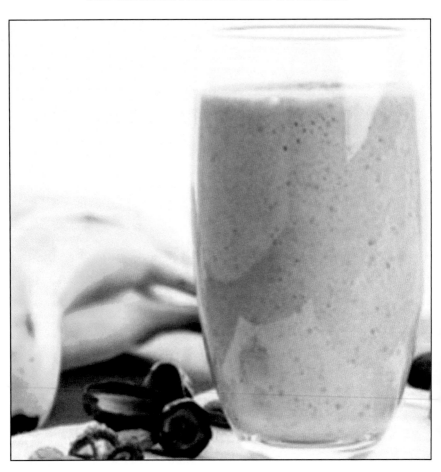

If you're ever craving butternut ice cream, then stop right here! This happy marriage of caramel, bananas, walnuts and coconut milk bring you something sweet, creamy and not too heavy. All without giving up being healthy. Decrease the liquid base and serve this thicker version as a dessert.

Prep Time: 5 min Serve: 2

Ingredients

- 2 cups spinach
- 2 cups sliced bananas
- 2 tablespoons caramel sauce
- 2 tablespoons walnuts
- 1 cup light coconut milk
- 1 cup non-dairy milk (soy, oat, almond, hemp or rice)

Directions

Put spinach, coconut milk and non-dairy milk into a blender. Blend until thoroughly mixed. Add bananas, caramel and walnuts. Blend until smooth. Pour into a tall glass and serve.

Why This is Good For You

- Low in cholesterol
- Low in sodium
- High in potassium
- High in vitamin B6
- Very high in vitamin C

Nutrition Facts

Calories 255, Calories from Fat 13, Total Fat 1.4g, Saturated Fat Trans Fat 0.0g, Cholesterol 4mg, Sodium 47mg, Potassium 621mg, Total Carbohydrates 34.0g, Dietary Fiber 3.7g, Sugars 20.4g, Protein 4.7g.

37. Tropical Green Blast

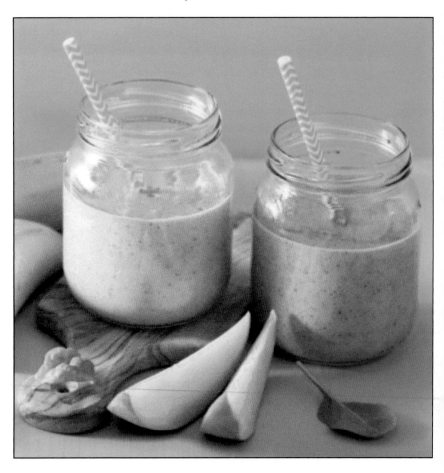

This simplified version of #10 will still blast your hair back when you're in a morning rush. Use frozen mangoes and pineapples to make this recipe a tropical breeze. A bold vitamin-loaded combination that is light and crisp, yet fruity.

Prep Time: 5 min, Serve: 2

Ingredients

- 4 cups spinach leaves
- 2 cups diced banana
- 1 cup diced ripe (or frozen) mangoes
- 1/2 cup ripe (or frozen) pineapple chunks
- 1/2 cup orange juice

Directions

Put spinach, banana, mango, pineapple and orange juice in the blender. Blend until ingredients are mixed.

Why This is Good For You

- Very low in sodium
- Very high in vitamin A
- Very high in vitamin C

Nutrition Facts

Calories 277, Sodium 31mg, Carbohydrates 97g, Dietary Fiber 4g, Sugars 83g, Protein 2g.

38. Green Lime Pie Smoothie

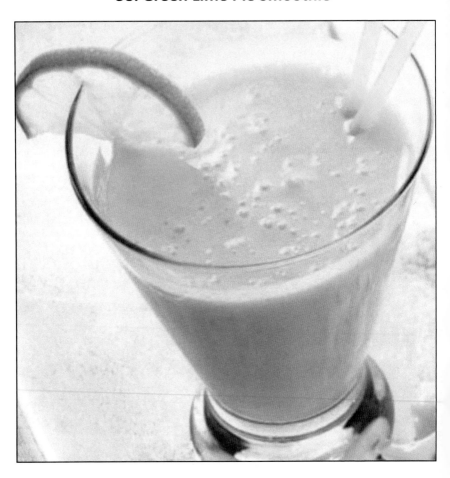

What do you get if you mix it up with bananas, lime zest, almond butter and a pitted date? You get a taste of key-lime pie, with none of the guilt. Feel free to use this as a dessert substitute, just adjust the sweetness to taste with some honey.

Prep Time: 5 min, Serve: 2

Ingredients

- 4 tablespoons lime juice
- 2 teaspoons lime zest
- 2 cups sliced ripe bananas
- 1/2 teaspoon pure vanilla extract
- 2 tablespoons almond butter (try sunflower butter)
- 4 cups shredded spinach leaves
- 2 whole pitted dates
- 2 cups unsweetened non-dairy milk (like soy or almond)
- 4 ice cubes
- crushed graham crackers for garnish

Directions

Put everything in a blender and whiz until smooth. Garnish with a lime and graham cracker crumbles.

Why This is Good For You

- No saturated fat
- No cholesterol
- No sodium
- High in vitamin C

Nutrition Facts

Calories 257, Calories from Fat 0, Total Fat 0g, Saturated Fat 0g, Polyunsaturated Fat 0g, Monounsaturated Fat 0g, Cholesterol 0mg, Sodium 0mg, Carbohydrates 52.6g, Dietary Fiber 5.8g, Sugars 51.8g, Protein 3.6g.

39. Spinach Fruit Medley

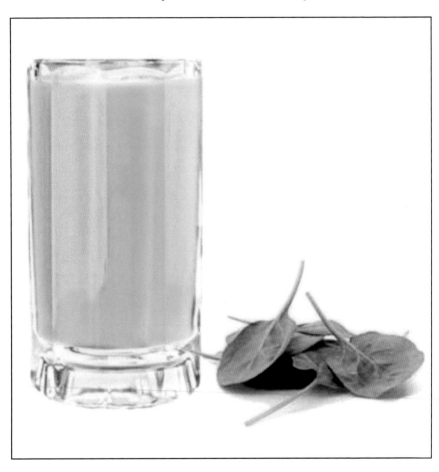

The Spinach Fruit Medley is everything you need in one glass for a quick morning start. The added yogurt produces a thick smoothie with a complex flavor. This one is so easy to drink that your children won't know it's healthy, so please don't tell them.

Prep Time: 5 min, Serve: 1

Ingredients

- 1 cup chopped spinach leaves
- 1/2 large whole orange
- 1/4 cup sliced bananas
- 1/6 cup frozen mixed berries
- 1/6 cup plain yogurt
- drizzle of agave nectar
- 1/2 cup ice cubes

Directions

Put all ingredients in a blender. Puree until smooth. Pour into glasses and serve immediately.

Why This is Good For You

- Low in cholesterol
- High in calcium
- High in manganese
- High in phosphorus
- High in potassium
- High in riboflavin
- Very high in vitamin A
- High in vitamin B6
- Very high in vitamin C

Nutrition Facts

Calories 195, Calories from Fat 23, Total Fat 2.6g, Saturated Fat 1.4g, Trans Fat 0.0g, Cholesterol 7mg, Sodium 111mg, Potassium 802mg, Total Carbohydrates 37.8g, Dietary Fiber 4.6g, Sugars 26.8g, Protein 8.9g.

40. Green Coconut Smoothie

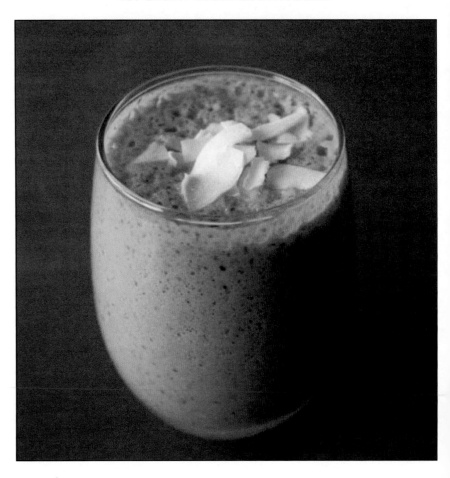

This deep-green treat has everything you need to keep going throughout a long day. Coconut meat and raw honey mingle with banana and kale to create a truly bar-raising smoothie. This one is drop, blend and drink. Don't forget some coconut on top!

Prep Time: 5 min, Serve: 2

Ingredients

- 2 cups chopped kale leaves
- 2 cups sliced ripe bananas
- 2 teaspoons raw honey
- 2 cups coconut meat
- 2 cups coconut water
- 1 cup ice cubes

Directions

In a blender, mix all ingredients until smooth. Pour into a glass and garnish with extra coconut meat.

Why This is Good For You

- Low in sodium
- High in calcium
- Very high in vitamin A
- Very high in vitamin C

Nutrition Facts

Calories 143, Calories from Fat 13, Total Fat 1.4g, Saturated Fat 1.3g, Trans Fat 0.0g, Sodium 34mg, Potassium 431mg, Total Carbohydrates 32.9g, Dietary Fiber 1.8g, Sugars 27.2g, Protein 1.1g.

41. Fig and Ginger Blast

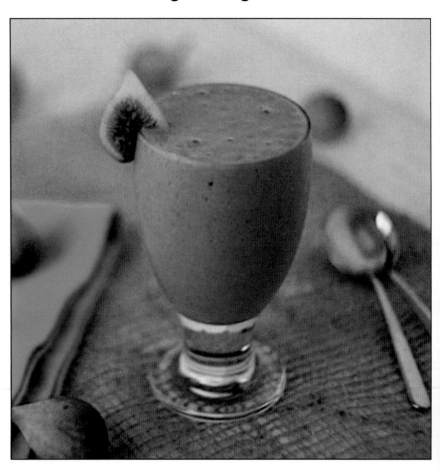

Spinach, figs, ginger and dates. Smooth with a full-bodied flavor, anything made with fig proves that no good fruit ever goes out of style. People have been eating figs since about 9,000 B.C. That's 6,000 years longer than people have been living in cities. But that young upstart Ginger didn't see wide use until the Roman times. This is how to kick it old school.

Prep Time: 5 min, Serve: 2

Ingredients

- 2 cups spinach
- 2 cups figs (about 8 medium sized fruits)
- 1 tablespoon chopped ginger
- 4 whole pitted dates (pre-soaked)
- 1 cup distilled water
- 2 cups ice cubes

Directions

In a blender, add spinach and water. Blend until smooth. Add all remaining ingredients and process until blended smoothly.

Why This is Good For You

- Very low in sodium
- High in dietary fiber
- High in vitamin
- A Very high in vitamin C

Nutrition Facts

Calories 352, Calories from Fat 104, Total Fat 16.3g, Saturated Fat 2.0g, Trans Fat 0.0g, Sodium 31mg Potassium, 1225mg, Total Carbohydrates 73.5g, Dietary Fiber 17.9g, Sugars 48.9g, Protein 8.7g.

42. Apple Broccoli Dream

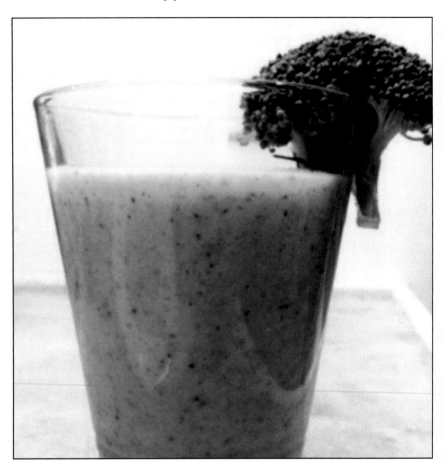

Get moving in the morning with this simple recipe that packs not only great taste but also a nice zip of energy. This wonderful blend is a graceful pairing of fruits and vegetables waltzing across your tongue, garbed in the finery that is vitamins and minerals.

Prep Time: 5 min, Serve: 1

Ingredients

- 1/2 cup shredded romaine lettuce
- 1/4 cup broccoli heads
- 1 medium sized apple
- 1/4 orange
- 1/4 cup distilled water
- 1/2 cup ice cubes

Directions

Rinse greens under running water. Peel and core apple. Cut into 1-inch cubes. Peel orange. Remove seeds and separate into segments. Put all ingredients in a blender. Blend on high speed until thoroughly combined. Pour into a glass and serve.

Why This is Good For You

- Low in cholesterol
- High in calcium
- High in manganese
- Very high in vitamin A
- Very high in vitamin C

Nutrition Facts

Calories 126, Calories from Fat 21, Total Fat 2.3g, Saturated Fat 1.2g, Trans Fat 0.0g, Cholesterol 4mg, Sodium 79mg, Potassium 359mg, Total Carbohydrates 16.4g, Dietary Fiber 2.6g, Sugars 12.7g, Protein 10.4g.

43. Summer Salad Smoothie

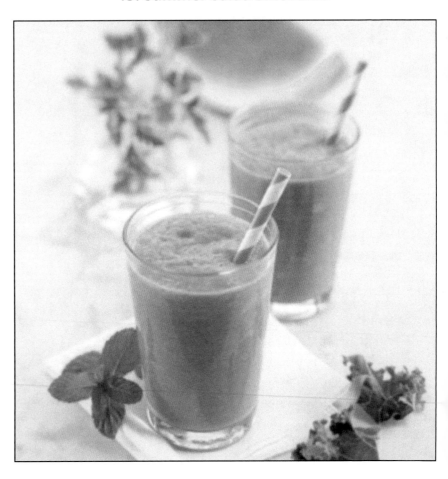

Need to cool down after a tough workout or a hot day at the beach? Did someone say pool party? Snap up a savory low-cal, citrus-infused Summer Salad Smoothie. Peppermint-herb is an excellent source of minerals like potassium, calcium, iron, manganese and magnesium.

Prep Time: 10 min, Serve: 2

Ingredients

- 20 leaves of mint
- 20 leaves of sweet basil
- 20 leaves of cilantro
- 4 cups watermelon chunks
- 1 small avocado fruit
- 1 cup cucumber slices
- Juice of 1 lime fruit
- 1 cup distilled water

Directions

Remove seeds from watermelon before cutting into chunks. Scoop out flesh from the avocado fruit. Slice cucumbers into half-inch thickness. Put all ingredients in a blender in this order: mint, basil, coriander, water, watermelon, avocado, cucumber, lime juice. Blend on high speed until smooth. Pour into a tall glass and serve.

Why This is Good For You

- Low in saturated fat
- No cholesterol
- Very low in sodium
- High in potassium
- Very high in vitamin A
- Very high in vitamin C

Nutrition Facts

Calories 46, Calories from Fat 2, Total Fat 0.2g, Saturated Fat 0.1g, Polyunsaturated Fat 0.1g, Monounsaturated Fat 0.1g, Cholesterol 0mg, Sodium 2mg, Potassium 171.21mg, Carbohydrates 11.6g, Dietary Fiber 0.6g, Sugars 9.5g Protein 0.9g.

44. Arugula Lettuce and Pear Rock

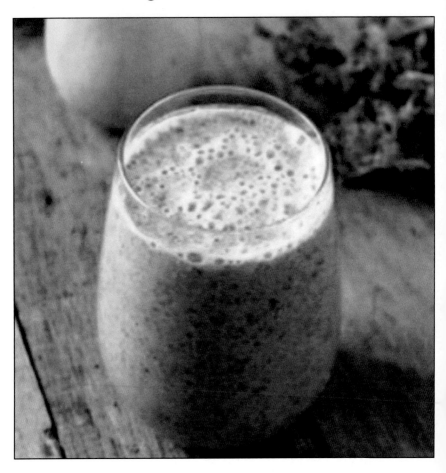

For the discerning connoisseur, try this little gem. Arugula lettuce thrown in with bananas, pears, hemp seeds and raspberries. This light and fruity beverage probably brings you everything your diet has been missing while keeping an appetizing appearance. You know you've made it correctly when it looks like the gemstone aventurine. It's so packed with minerals that it even looks like one.

Prep Time: 5 min, Serve: 2

Ingredients

- 2 bananas, 2 pears
- 2 tablespoons hulled hemp seed
- 1 cup of frozen raspberries
- 5 cups pure water
- small bunch of arugula leaves
- Liquid Stevia (or any sweetener) to taste

Directions

Add enough water so that all ingredients are covered. Blend well.

Why This is Good For You

- Low in saturated fat
- No cholesterol
- Very high in calcium
- Very high in dietary fiber
- Very high in iron
- Very high in manganese
- Very high in magnesium
- High in pantothenic acid
- Very high in phosphorus
- Very high in potassium
- High in riboflavin
- High in thiamin
- Very high in vitamin A
- High in vitamin B6
- Very high in vitamin C
- High in zinc

Nutrition Facts

Calories 300, Calories from Fat 1, Total Fat 0.1g, Saturated Fat 0g, Polyunsaturated Fat 0g, Monounsaturated Fat 0g, Cholesterol 0mg, Sodium 3mg, Potassium 36.9mg, Carbohydrates 0.4g, Dietary Fiber 0.2g, Sugars 0.2g, Protein 0.3g.

45. Carrot Ginger Twist

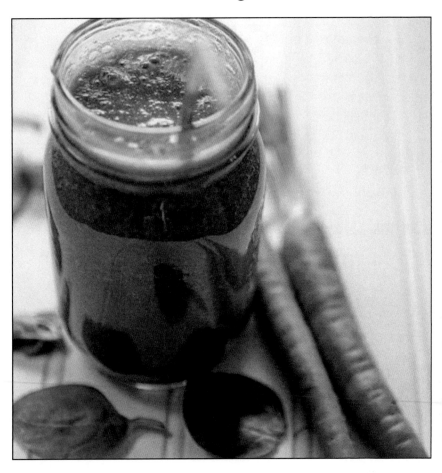

It's often said that carrots are great for your eyes, but the Carrot Ginger Twist is great for everything. The carrots natural sweetness is complemented by just a bite of spice. An ideal choice to get that extra bit of zest that you've been looking for.

Prep Time: 5 min, Serve: 2

Ingredients

- 1 bunch of carrots with some of its greens
- 1 avocado
- 1/2 lemon
- 1/3 inch fresh ginger
- Pinch of sea salt and cayenne pepper

Directions

Put all ingredients in your juicer. Add clean water to cover all ingredients. Blend. Drink immediately.

Why This is Good For You

- Very low in saturated fat
- Low in sodium
- High in dietary fiber
- High in manganese
- High in potassium
- Very high in vitamin A
- Very high in vitamin C

Nutrition Facts

Calories 174, Calories from Fat 3, Total Fat 0.3g, Saturated Fat 0.1g, Trans Fat 0.0g, Sodium 86mg, Potassium 949mg, Total Carbohydrates 42.7g, Dietary Fiber 6.0g, Sugars 26.8g, Protein 3.3g.

46. The Pumpkin Smooth BOO, Charlie Brown!

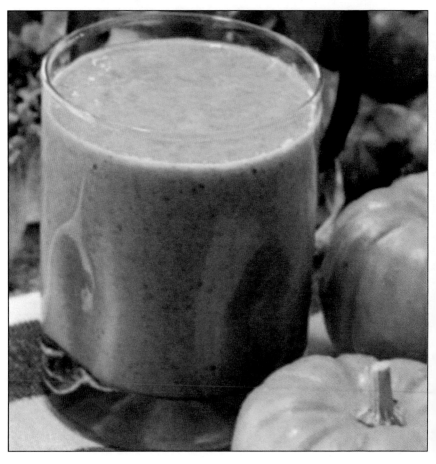

Guaranteed to be a major hit when the leaves begin to change, The Pumpkin Smooth delivers plenty of protein with flavors inspired by pumpkin. This concoction is on the thicker side and carries the savory taste of autumn. Its complement of vitamins A, C and E spell this smoothie out for the ace it really is. Drink it while you wait for the Great Pumpkin to rise.

Prep Time: 5 min, Serve: 2

Ingredients

- 1 cup pure canned pumpkin
- 2 cups fresh or frozen mango
- 6 tablespoons cashews
- 1 teaspoon vanilla extract.
- 1 teaspoon cinnamon
- 4 cups baby spinach
- 16 ounces unsweetened almond milk

Directions

Put all ingredients into blender and blend until smooth.

Why This is Good For You

- Low in saturated fat
- No cholesterol
- Very high in calcium
- High in dietary fiber
- High in iron
- Very high in manganese
- High in magnesium
- High in potassium
- Very high in vitamin A
- High in vitamin B6
- Very high in vitamin C
- Very high in vitamin E

Nutrition Facts

Calories 191, Calories from Fat 28, Total Fat 3.1g, Saturated Fat 0.3g, Trans Fat 0.0g, Cholesterol 0mg, Sodium 235mg, Potassium 1180mg, Total Carbohydrates 40.0g, Dietary Fiber 9.4g, Sugars 18.3g, Protein 5.2g.

47. Cucumber Beet Smoothies

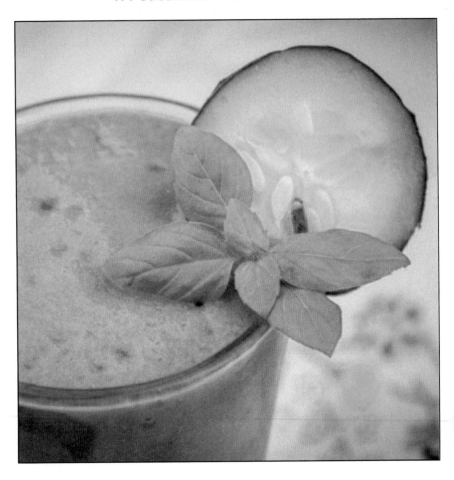

Ginger, beets and cucumbers combine to bring you a fresh taste of India. Raw beets are an excellent source of folates that go along wonderfully with the fiber from celery. Garnish with a leaf to brighten it up. If you use traditional red beets, your smoothie will be more of a brown color.

Prep Time: 5 min, Serve: 2

Ingredients

- 1 golden (or red) beet root
- 2 cucumbers
- 4 sticks of celery
- 6 carrots
- 2 red apples
- an inch of ginger

Directions

Put all Ingredients in a blender and blend until smooth.

Why This is Good For You

- Low in saturated fat
- No cholesterol
- High in dietary fiber
- Very high in manganese
- High in magnesium
- High in potassium
- Very high in vitamin A
- Very high in vitamin C

Nutrition Facts

Calories 111, Calories from Fat 20, Total Fat 2.2g, Saturated Fat 0.2g, Trans Fat 0.0g, Cholesterol 0mg, Sodium 74mg, Potassium 514mg, Total Carbohydrates 23.9g, Dietary Fiber 5.3g, Sugars 15.7g, Protein 3.1g.

48. Avocado Carrot Basil Smoothie

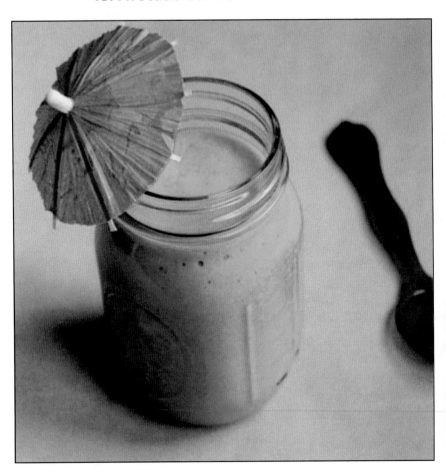

This smoothie is very easy to make and packed full of healthy foods. The added basil leaves give this smoothie a whole new dimension of flavor. Combined with all the vitamins and minerals from its ingredients, this recipe is a "complete package".

Prep Time: 5 min Serve: 2

Ingredients

- 4 carrots
- 1 apple
- 1 cup avocado
- 1 basil leaves
- 1 orange wedge (or ½ cup orange juice)
- 1 cup kale

Directions

Extract juice from carrot and apple in a juicer. Transfer to a blender and add the avocado and a handful of basil leaves. Blend until smooth and squeeze orange.

Why This is Good For You

- No cholesterol
- Low in sodium
- High in dietary fiber
- High in potassium
- Very high in vitamin A
- High in vitamin C

Nutrition Facts

Calories 408, Calories from Fat 100, Total Fat 22.2g, Saturated Fat 3.2g, Trans Fat 0.0g, Cholesterol 0mg, Sodium 180mg, Potassium 1648mg, Total Carbohydrates 55.5g, Dietary Fiber 20.1g 80%, Sugars 27.0g, Protein 5.6g.

49. Banana-Walnut Heaven

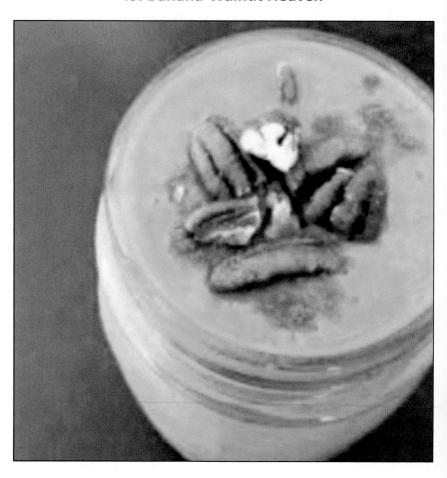

This is a delicious and healthy smoothie of milk, honey, vanilla and walnuts that combine to create a dense, dessert-worthy shake. Add in bananas and you simply can't go wrong. This one is a one-step recipe, so it's great when you're pressed for time, especially when you need a quick pick-me-up.

Prep Time: 5 min, Serve: 4

Ingredients

- 4 cups skim milk
- 2 large bananas
- 2 tablespoons honey
- 1/2 teaspoon vanilla extract
- Handful walnut pieces, extra for garnish
- 1 cup of chopped kale

Directions

Blend all ingredients together. Garnish with walnuts.

Why This is Good For You

- Very low in cholesterol
- Low in sodium
- High in manganese
- High in magnesium
- High in phosphorus
- High in vitamin C

Nutrition Facts

Calories 171, Calories from Fat 58, Total Fat 6.5g, Saturated Fat 0.8g, Trans Fat 0.0g, Sodium 98mg, Potassium 258mg, Total Carbohydrates 25.0g, Dietary Fiber 2.2g, Sugars 17.8g, Protein 2.9g.

50. Peach Chia Smoothie

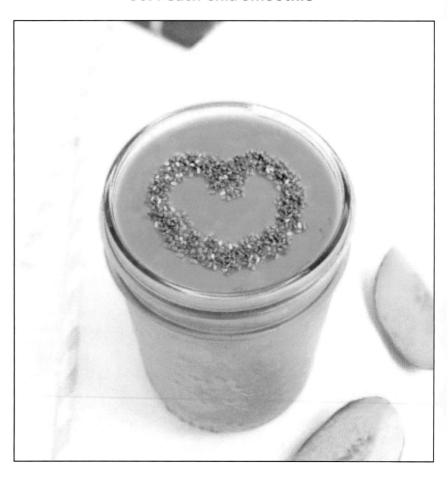

We end our journey with this delectable fruit blend smoothie that is sprinkled with a little love. Life is too short to live it unhealthily. Be bold. Try new things, like chia seeds.

Prep Time: 5 min, Serve: 2

Ingredients

- 2 peaches, pitted or frozen slices
- 4 cups romaine leaves
- 4 tablespoons chia seeds
- 1 frozen diced banana
- 1 orange
- 1/2 cup plain yogurt

Directions

Enter all ingredients in a blender and blend until smooth. Sprinkle heart design onto smoothie.

Why This is Good For You

- No saturated fat
- No cholesterol
- No sodium
- High in dietary fiber
- Very high in vitamin A

Nutrition Facts

Calories 120, Calories from Fat 9, Total Fat 1g, Saturated Fat 0g, Polyunsaturated Fat 0g, Monounsaturated Fat 0g, Cholesterol 0mg, Sodium 0mg, Potassium 330.01mg, Carbohydrates 27g, Dietary Fiber 4g, Sugars 24g, Protein 2g.

Conclusion

Two weeks have passed since the beginning of Sabrina's new morning routine. While she is six pounds lighter, it is the difference in her energy level and outlook that brings her the most joy and pride. Waking up in the morning is less of a struggle - in fact, she hasn't even used the snooze button on her alarm clock a single time in the past week. Every morning she wakes up feeling rested and ready for the rest of her day. Sabrina even notices that work is both easier and more productive. She often finds herself amazed at how such a small change like adding green smoothies to her mornings has made such a major difference in her life. Over the weeks, she finds an affinity for Raspberry Ripple and the Blueberry Flourish Smoothie. She usually has one in the morning, but nothing else in her diet or routine has changed, although she often feels as if it has. It is wonderful being on a diet that does not require obsessing over calories. Sabrina muses on how easy it is while sipping on her Cranberry Kickstarter. Taking a moment to bask in the flavor, she wonders if perhaps she has found a new favorite. This new diet seems to be infectious: on the first weekend of Sabrina's new diet, her best friend decided to join her. Having never used a blender before, she switched it on and walked off to another room. They spent the rest of the morning cleaning Carrot Ginger Twist off the ceiling, but at least the smell was a welcome one. Overall, Sabrina is proud of the progress that she has made. Just a few weeks ago, she never imagined that changes so slight and easy would set her on the path to health. Smoothies save her time, bring her energy and provide her with a great breakfast each morning. She tells her friends, her workmates, her family. And she makes certain to remind them to keep a hand on the blender lid.

Other Book by Dr. Duc Vuong

Meditate to Lose Weight: A Guide For A Slimmer Healthier You

Healthy Eating on a Budget: A How-To Guide

Eating Healthy for Kids: A How-To Guide

Healthy Green Smoothies: 50 Easy Recipes That Will Change Your Life

Big-Ass Salads: 31 Easy Recipes For Your Healthy Month

Weight Loss Surgery Success: Dr. V's A-Z Steps For Losing Weight And Gaining Enlightenment

The Ultimate Gastric Sleeve Success: A Practical Patient Guide

Lap-Band Rescue: Revisit. Rethink. Revise.

Duc-It-Up: 366 Tips To Improve Your Life

Made in the USA
Monee, IL
21 January 2020